SELENIUM AROUND THE WORLD

Large-scale studies in China and Finland, involving thousands—sometimes tens of thousands—of subjects, have demonstrated conclusively the protective role of the trace mineral selenium in both cancer and heart disease, and each new research effort in the United States and other countries adds to the evidence. Dr. Passwater, a pioneer selenium proponent, presents the latest information on the lifesaving properties of this little-known nutrient.

SELENIUM UPDATE

HOW IT PROTECTS AGAINST CANCER, HEART DISEASE, ARTHRITIS AND AGING

by Richard A. Passwater, Ph.D.

Keats Publishing, Inc. ✶ New Canaan, Connecticut

Selenium Update is not intended as medical advice. Its intention is solely informational and educational. Please consult a medical or health professional should the need for one be indicated.

SELENIUM UPDATE

ISBN: 0-87983-393-9

Printed in the United States of America

Good Health Guides are published by
Keats Publishing, Inc.
27 Pine Street (Box 876)
New Canaan, Connecticut 06840

Contents

INTRODUCTION

Selenium is a trace element (mineral) that is vital to your health. Just like the minerals iron and calcium, it is needed in your diet or you will die of malnutrition. If you do get some—but not enough—selenium in your diet, you won't develop outright malnutrition, but will instead have greater chances of getting cancer, heart disease, and arthritis and of experiencing accelerated aging. Now there is exciting and strong evidence the optimal selenium intake will prevent or reduce the incidence of many deadly diseases. This book tells the dramatic selenium story and explains how proper selenium nutrition can safely improve and lengthen your life.

BACKGROUND

It is gratifying to see that the research that I performed in the early 1960s showing that selenium increases the life span and prevents cancer has now been accepted by most scientists and physicians involved in those areas of research. Also, it has been exciting to see that researchers have expanded animal studies to show that selenium is protective against heart disease, as well as protective and sometimes curative in arthritis and other diseases. Selenium is not a wonder drug. These diseases are all dependent on a common factor called a "free radical," and selenium is a nutrient that stimulates the body's defense against free radicals.

While "free radical" is not quite yet a household word, the term is in common use among the most knowledgeable of those interested in improving their lives with optimal nutrition. Our interest in free radicals is due to their high reactivity with vital body components. It is not necessary that we understand what free radicals are or how they do their damage, but it does help if we have a "word picture" conceptual use of the term. A simplified definition of free radicals is given in Box 1.

The pace of research on selenium and health is very brisk right now, and many scientists and research physicians are entering the field because of the strength of the research results and the promise of even more health benefits to come. Now scientists often start their investigations without thoroughly reviewing the works of the pioneers that preceded them, including Coombs, Schrauzer, Scott, Schwarz, Shamberger, Spallholtz, Tappel and myself. Of these selenium pioneers, only Schrauzer, Shamberger and I experimented with selenium as an anticancer nutrient. If the newcomers, with their broad array of talent and sophisticated skills, would dig out the published studies of the 1960s and early 1970s, they would find that much of what they are publishing as new discoveries has already been published—admittedly, however, based on the less sophisticated experimental techniques of those times.

As newcomers enter the field, they find that there are hundreds of studies over two decades involving thousands of people and laboratory animals. My first scientific presentation of my 1960s research showing that selenium in synergistic combination with other nutrient antioxidants (anti-free radical compounds) slowed the aging process in laboratory animals was at the twenty-third Gerontological Society Meeting in Toronto in October 1970. A confirmation of the anti-free radical power of my synergistic formulation was reported in *Pathological Aspects of Cell Membranes* (Academic Press, 1971) by Dr. A. L. Tappel of the University of California at Davis. My first scientific presentation of how selenium and other nutrient antioxidants in synergistic combination prevented cancer appeared in the magazine *American Laboratory* in May 1973. Earlier presentations of my research were in patent applications and news articles. (See Box 2 for a bibliography of reports on my early research on this topic.)

These studies were small-scale experiments involving small laboratory animals. Few scientists thought that the results would apply to humans in the real world. Few scientists wanted to risk their reputations and future funding by conducting the needed clinical trials with only laboratory animal studies and a strange new theory about "free-radical pathology" as the supporting evidence.

The good news is that we pioneers kept hammering away,

BOX 2

Bibliography of the author's early publications on anticancer activity of selenium

In the scientific press:

1. *The Gerontologist*, 10(3):28, Oct. 1970
2. *Chem. & Eng. News* 48:17 (Oct. 26, 1970). Followup: May 10, 1971
3. *Geriatric Focus*, March-April 1971
4. *American Lab* 3(4):36-40, April 1971
5. *American Lab* 3(5):21-25, May 1971
6. *American Lab* 5(6):10-22, May 1973
7. *American Lab* 8(4) 32-47, Aug. 1976

U.S. Patent Numbers 39140 and 97011, and patents in various other countries.

In the general interest press:

1. *Washington Daily News* p. 5, Sept. 15, 1970
2. *Prevention* 23(12) 104-110, Dec. 1971
3. Reuters News Agency report, Oct. 23, 1970
4. *Ladies' Home Journal* 70, 129-131, July 1971
5. Kugler, H., *Slowing the Aging Process*, Pyramid, NY, 1973
6. Rosenfeld, A., *Prolongevity*, Knopf, NY, 1976

expanding our experiments, lecturing our colleagues, and daring somebody to prove us wrong. Unfortunately, some of us were often chastised or labeled "quacks" by those not able to understand free-radical pathology. Therefore, we had to become "activists" to bring this important research before as many scientists as we could. The great news is that the new scientists who entered the field brought with them new skills and capabilities that produced different kinds of evidence that selenium did prevent cancer, heart disease and arthritis and did slow the aging process. Here is a look at the exciting new evidence involving clinical trials, epidemiological studies and laboratory studies. You don't have to be a biochemist to understand how strong the evidence is.

A brief explanation as to how selenium prevents cancer is given in the diagram below.

Properties and functions of selenium that may be related to its anticarcinogenic action

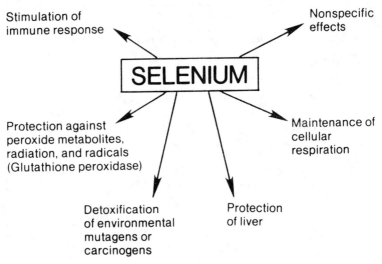

Source: Schrauzer, G. 1978. *Inorganic and Nutritional Aspects of Cancer.* New York: Plenum Press, p. 330.

CANCER

Selenium prevents cancer. There is even evidence that selenium may help cure cancer. Selenium by itself can't protect all people from all types of cancer, but it definitely reduces the incidences of all types of cancer studied so far in large populations. Some individuals may have genetic weaknesses, or be so undernourished that their immune system can't function, or be so overwhelmed with chemicals that cause cancer, that they don't have a chance. However, most people are not so unfortunate, and selenium will reduce their risk of getting cancer by strengthening their immune system and protecting their vital cell components against free-radical attack.

Through hundreds of laboratory studies, case-controlled clinical studies and epidemiological studies, it has been consistently demonstrated that the better the selenium nutriture of a person, the less chance of cancer. The evidence for a prophylactic role for selenium is without a doubt stronger than for any other factor, including the nutrient beta-carotene, dietary fiber, crucifers or any other food factor recommended as potential cancer-preventive agents by the American Cancer Society, National Cancer Institute, and other official bodies.

The evidence includes the following types of study:

Clinical: prospective, retrospective

Epidemiological: blood levels, food intake, soils

Animal: life span, spontaneous cancer; carcinogen-induced (dietary, contact); virus-induced (not inoculated, inoculated); transplanted cancer tissue; inoculated cancer cells

Therapeutic

The protective action of selenium against every type of cancer studied has been demonstrated regardless of whether the cancer-causing agents have been introduced in the laboratory or naturally, chemically or virally induced, inoculated or transplanted.

The clinical confirmation that cancer probability correlates inversely with a person's blood selenium content (the higher the selenium, the less chance of cancer) was shown epidemiologically in the 1970s by Dr. Raymond Shamberger and clinically in the *New England Journal of Medicine* by Harvard's Dr. W. C. Willet and colleagues in 1983.

There is no need to review the hundreds of tests. Let's just start with six recent studies that should catch your attention. Here is a brief summary of the major points they make (the studies are discussed in greater detail in the next section, and identified here by the name of the principal author in parenthesis):

1. Considering selenium blood levels alone, those persons in the *lowest* fifth of all blood selenium levels *have twice the incidence of cancer* as those in the highest fifth (Willett, 1983).

2. Total cancer mortality is *three times higher* in persons having *blood selenium values below a certain value* than the incidence of cancer in those above this value (Yu, 1985).

3. Considering selenium blood levels alone, those persons in the *lowest* tenth of all blood selenium levels *have six times the incidence of* cancer as those in the highest tenth (Clark, 1984).

4. Both selenium and vitamin E are needed together to prevent cancer (Horvath, 1983).

5. When considering both selenium and vitamin E blood levels, those persons in the lowest third of blood vitamin E level and also having a low blood selenium level had *more than eleven times the incidence of* cancer as those in the upper two-thirds of blood vitamin E and selenium levels (Salonen, 1985).

6. Still another researcher concludes that "selenium should be considered not only as a preventive, but also as a therapeutic agent in cancer treatment and may act additively or synergistically with drug and X-ray treatments" (Milner, 1984).

Now where have I heard those words before?

I hope those studies have your attention. The next section describes them in detail. The section also includes graphic illustration of several other studies indicating inverse relationship between cancer incidence and selenium intake. Figures 1 through 3 deal with the occurrence of cancer in the United States; Figure 4 relates selenium intake and breast cancer in several countries; Figure 5 shows the results of experiments with laboratory animals in which cancers were induced.

The epidemiological studies by themselves do not prove anything, but combining them with the clinical studies and laboratory experiments allows a valid conclusion to be inferred.

Figure 1. Zero cancer extrapolations

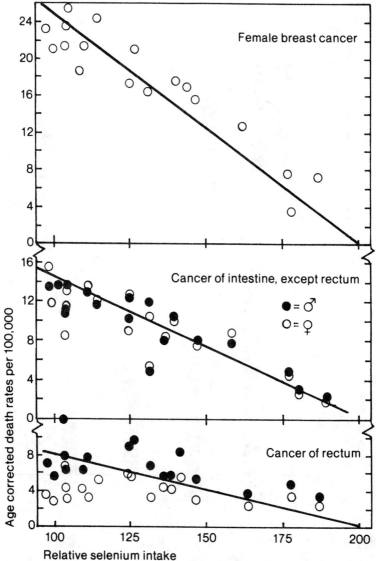

Source: Schrauzer, White, and Schneider, 1977. *Bioinorganic Chem.* 7:37.

Figures 2 and 3. Cancer death rate versus selenium level

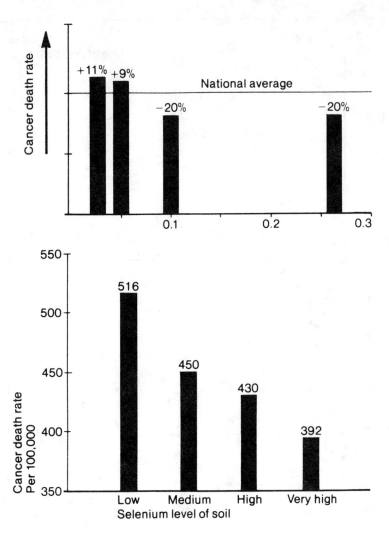

Sources: Passwater drawings based on data from Shamberger, R. and Frost, D. 1969. *Canadian Medical Association Journal* 100:682.

Figure 4. Relationship of selenium intake and breast cancer mortalities

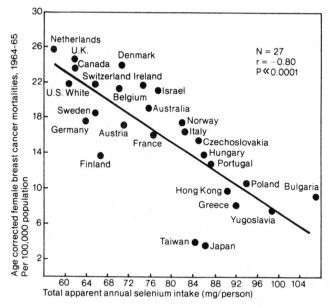

Source: Schrauzer, G., White, D. and Schneider, C. 1977.
Bioinorganic Chemistry, vol. 7, p. 36.

Figure 5. Protective effect of selenium against carcinogen-produced cancer in animals

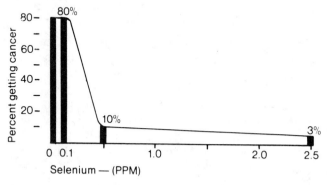

Source: Passwater drawing based on data from Harr, J., Exon, J., Whanger, P. and Weswig, P. 1972. *Clinical Toxicology* 5(2):187–94.

SIX STUDIES OF IMPORTANCE

The Willet Study

This study is of major importance not only for its research but for its influence. The Willett study was conducted by a well-respected group of researchers, and the work was done at major centers of learning: Harvard, Johns Hopkins, Duke, the University of Texas and other respected colleges and universities. The results were published in a major medical journal, rather than an obscure scientific periodical. Many physicians read of the importance of blood selenium levels and their relationship to cancer risk for the first time, thanks to this study.

In the Willett study, blood samples had been collected in 1973 from 4480 men from fourteen regions of the United States. At the time of collection of the blood samples, none of the men had detectable signs of cancer. The blood samples were preserved and stored for later analysis.

During the next five years, 111 cases of cancer were detected in the group. The researchers then retrieved the stored blood samples from these men, and from 210 other men who were selected because they matched the newly-developed cancer patients in age, sex, race and smoking history. The levels of several nutrients and other factors were compared between the men who developed cancer and those men who remained free of cancer.

One difference stood out as being highly significant. The risk of cancer for subjects in the lowest quintile (fifth) of blood selenium was twice that of subjects in the highest. (W. C. Willett et al., "Prediagnostic Serum Selenium and Risk of Cancer." *Lancet* II:130-4, July 16, 1983)

The Chinese Study

This study, examining the relationship between blood levels of selenium in 1458 healthy adults in 24 regions of China, was led by Dr. Shu-Yu Yu of the Cancer Institute of the Chinese Academy of Medical Sciences in Beijing. The researchers found that there was a statistically significant inverse correlation between age-adjusted cancer death rates and the selenium levels in the blood of local residents. In the areas with high selenium levels, there was significantly lower cancer mortality in both males and females. Total cancer mortality was three times higher in ares where mean blood selenium level was greater than 11 micrograms per deciliter of blood than where it was 8 micrograms per deciliter. (Shu-Yu Yu et al., "Regional Variation of Cancer Mortality Incidence and its Relation to Selenium Levels in China." *Biological Trace Element Research* 7:21-9, Jan.-Feb. 1985)

The Clark Study

Dr. Larry C. Clark and colleagues at Cornell determined the blood selenium levels in 240 skin cancer patients and compared the results to those from 103 apparently healthy persons living in low-selenium areas. The mean blood selenium level for the skin cancer patients was significantly lower than that of the apparently healthy individuals. After adjusting for age, sun damage to the skin, blood beta-carotene and vitamin A levels, and other factors, the incidence of skin cancer in those persons in the lowest decile (tenth) of blood selenium was 5.8 times as great as those in the highest decile. (L. C. Clark et al., "Plasma Selenium and Skin Neoplasms: A Case Controlled Study." *Nutrition and Cancer* (6:13-21, Jan.-Mar. 1984)

The Horvath Study

The preceding three studies have dealt with real people, but let's look at an important laboratory animal study for a moment. Most scientific experiments examine one variable at a time to study the effect of just that one variable. This reduces confusion from confounding factors. Yet the body is not a simple laboratory, it is a biologically complex mechanism that functions independently of science's effort to study it. While this booklet is written primarily about selenium, I want to stress that total nutrition is important. If you are grossly deficient in vitamin A or vitamin E, the correct amount of selenium will not make up for all the deficiencies.

However, there is more to the relationship than balanced total nutrition. There is a special synergistic relationship among all the antioxidant nutrients, but especially vitamin E and selenium. This has been the essence of my research and the basis for my patents and publications. In 1983, a sophisticated study was published by Drs. Paula Horvath and Clement Ip that clarified this synergistic relationship of vitamin E and selenium.

They found that vitamin E and selenium must both be present to prevent the proliferating phase of cancer. Their evidence indicates that it is not the amount of selenium-containing gluta-thione peroxidase that is critical but the amount of microsomal peroxidase activity, which is stimulated only by the presence of both vitamin E and selenium. (P. M. Horvath and C. Ip, "Synergistic Effect of Vitamin E and Selenium in the Chemoprevention of Mammary Carcinogenesis in Rats." *Cancer Research* 43:5335-41, Nov. 1983)

The message here is that scientists should not be studying the correlation between blood selenium levels alone and cancer but studying the blood levels of vitamin E and selenium together. Studying selenium alone, we do in fact find that there is a substantial reduction in cancer risk with the higher blood levels of selenium. But we find the same relationship with vitamin E and some types of cancer—the more vitamin E in the blood, the lower the incidence of cancer. As an example consider the report in the *British Journal of Cancer* (49:321-324, 1984) by Dr. N. J. Wald that showed that women in the lowest quintile of vitamin E levels had 5.2 times the risk of cancer as women in the highest. However, when a person's blood is rich in both vitamin E and selenium, the protection given that person is far more than that of adding the vitamin E protection and the selenium protection together.

If a person has a normal blood level of selenium, but is very deficient in vitamin E, that person will not have a good defense against cancer. Conversely, if a person is a little low in selenium—but well fortified with vitamin E—then that person may be more resistant to cancer.

Since the vitamin E blood level can affect the usefulness of selenium, researchers should be looking at the combined levels, not just a simple selenium level. Once researchers catch on to this relationship, we will see even more dramatic results. This becomes apparent in the next study.

The Finnish Study

Dr. Jukka Salonen and his colleagues at the University of Kuopio (Finland) have been studying over 12,000 Finns for several years. The study is known as the North Karelia Project. Four years after drawing blood samples from these 12,155 persons, 51 had died of cancer. They were matched by age, sex and smoking habits with others and their blood samples were compared.

In this study many factors were examined, but most important, both vitamin E and selenium levels of the blood were examined in combination. The relative risk of cancer mortality for the third of people with blood selenium levels below 47 micrograms per liter of blood compared to those with higher levels was 5.8 to 1. But of more importance is the finding that, for people with low selenium levels who also had vitamin E levels in the lowest of values, risk of death from *cancer compared to persons with both selenium and vitamin E levels in the upper two-thirds of values was 11.4 to 1.* (J. T. Salonen et al., "Risk of Cancer in Relation to Serum Concentrations of Selenium and Vitamins A and E." *British Medical Journal* 290:417-20, Feb. 9, 1985)

The Milner Review

Dr. John A. Milner of the University of Illinois has been studying selenium and cancer prevention for more than a decade. Most of Dr. Milner's studies involve transplanting or inoculating cancer cells into mice receiving different levels of selenium. He has found that selenium inhibits the development of such cancer.

Dr. Milner's conclusion is that selenium should be considered not only as a preventive but also as a therapeutic agent in cancer treatment. There is evidence, which will be presented here later, that selenium may act additively or synergistically with drug and X-ray treatments. (J.A. Milner, "Selenium and the Transplantable Tumor." *Journal of Agricultural and Food Chemistry* 32:436-42, May-June 1984)

Nutrition Reviews Brings the News to the Nutritionists

These six studies will eventually have a major impact on cancer research. However, the subject is still new to most researchers and especially so to those who hold fast to the notion that diet and cancer are not related. To begin to educate such "old-line" nutritionists, the conservative nutrition journal *Nutrition Reviews* published an issue devoted to the topic.

Drs. Gerald Combs and Larry Clark of Cornell present an excellent review of selenium's protective roles against cancer in the November 1985 issue of *Nutrition Reviews*. Their review article is entitled "Can Dietary Selenium Modify Cancer Risk?" and the evidence that they present is quite convincing. (43:325-331) They provide 97 references for the serious scholar to pursue. Most scientists who bother to read those 97 reference articles will become selenium fans, but there are five times that many in the literature, and they should be read to really understand the depth of the research that supports the hypothesis.

Since *Nutrition Reviews* is widely read by nutritional scientists—and keep in mind that nutritionists usually are not regular readers of the journals on cancer research—the importance of selenium may finally be appreciated by nutritionists.

Blood Level of Selenium Is Critical

One important aspect of selenium research is that blood or hair levels of selenium are of major importance. It is not just simply a matter of what foods one eats, or how much selenium is present in those foods. Foods vary greatly in their selenium content, and just as important, food selenium varies greatly in its availability to the body. Sometimes the food selenium is present in a form more readily assimilated than other forms, and sometimes the selenium is "tied up" with other compounds such as mercury and is unavailable to the body. This is why selenium supplements are important, as they are bioavailable and in measured doses. The importance of blood levels will become clearer in the following section concerning the use of selenium in cancer therapy.

CANCER THERAPY

In the early 1970s, when it was clear that optimal intake of selenium was protective against cancer in laboratory animals, Dr. Gerhard Schrauzer of the University of California at San Diego and I called for clinical trials to test for this capability in humans. Dr. Schrauzer had completed a series of experiments that showed that optimal selenium intake could reduce the natural occurrence of breast cancer in mice by nearly 90 percent to only 12 percent of the normal cancer rate. (G. Schrauzer and D. Ishmael, *Annals of Clinical Laboratory Science* 4:441-7, 1974). He told the National Cancer Institute in 1978 that the key to cancer prevention lies in assuring adequate selenium intake.

Dr. Schrauzer stated in a 1978 article in *Family Circle* that if every woman in America started taking selenium (supplements) today or had a high-selenium diet, within a few years the breast cancer rate would decline drastically. He also remarked that if a breast cancer patient has low selenium levels in her blood, her tendency to develop metastases (other tumors) is increased, her possibility for survival is diminished, and her prognosis in general is poorer than if she had normal levels.

These observations were based on the experience of a group led by Dr. K. McConnell and may have been what set several surgeons looking to see if better selenium and other nutrient antioxidant nourishment would improve patients' chances of recovery. And guess what—they do.

Recent results in treating cancer patients with selenium have been astonishing! However, there are successful reports in the medical literature going back to the 1950s that were missed even by the selenium pioneers working with laboratory animals. In 1956 four leukemia patients were given an organic compound that contains selenium called slenocystine. In all four cases, a rapid decrease of the total leukocyte count was observed, as well as a reduction in spleen size. The most striking results were obtained in the cases of acute leukemia. (A. Weisberger and L. Suhrland, *Blood* 11:19, 1956)

In 1975, as referred to above, Dr. McConnell noticed a link between the survival times of 110 cancer patients and their blood selenium levels. Dr. McConnell and his colleagues concluded that those patients with the lowest blood selenium levels were more likely to have far-spreading cancer, multiple tumors located in different organ systems and multiple recurrences. (K. McConnell, W. Broghamer, A. Blotcky and O. Hurt, *Journal of Nutrition* 105:1026-31, 1975; W. Broghamer, K. McConnell and A. Blotcky, *Cancer* 37:1384, 1976)

Conversely, those patients whose cancers were confined and who rarely suffered recurrences all had higher (but still subnormal) selenium levels. These same researchers determined in 1978 that the blood selenium levels of breast cancer patients were lower than in women in the same age brackets without breast cancer. (K. McConnell, *Advances in Nutrition Research*, vol. 2, ed. by H. Draper. New York: Plenum Press, 1979, p. 225)

Several surgeons and oncologists are now using selenium and other antioxidant nutrients to successfully treat cancer. However, since such adjunct nutritional therapy may be considered "experimental" in the legal sense in the case of malpractice suits, these doctors do not wish to be publicized. Also, there is that ever-present concern among doctors not to appear to be food faddists or quacks by using food supplements in new ways. But physicians should now recognize that the wealth of data and truth is on the side that selenium helps the body overcome cancer and it is criminal *not* to use selenium supplements as adjunct therapy. For the good of mankind it is now time for all of these researchers to put their fears behind them and speak up—and let their results do the talking.

In 1983 I reported in my book *Cancer and Its Nutritional Therapies: Updated Edition* (Keats Publishing), that Dr. R. Donaldson of the St. Louis Veterans Administration Hospital orally reported his results to the National Cancer Institute (May 9, 1983) and the Annual Meeting of VA Surgeons (1980). These reports showed remarkable results for the use of selenium in treating terminally ill cancer patients and emphasize the need for further large-scale investigation of such use. Dr. Donaldson's studies and their results have not yet been published in the professional literature, perhaps because they are considered preliminary, but the bare facts of this work are important enough to merit mention here.

At the time of Dr. Donaldson's presentation to the National Cancer Institute, he had 140 patients enrolled in his study. According to the data that I have, all the patients who entered his study were certified as being terminally ill by two physicians after receiving the appropriate conventional therapy for their particular cancer. Some of the patients who entered the program with only weeks to live were alive and well after four years, and with no signs or symptoms of cancer. Not all patients were cured, but all had reduction in tumor size and pain. It is unfortunate that they did not receive the selenium until they were pronounced incurable. This research may well change cancer therapy in the future.

It is important to realize that the dramatic improvements did not occur until sufficient selenium was ingested to bring the patient's blood selenium level up to normal. Sometimes this could be achieved in a few weeks with 200–600 micrograms of selenium per day, while other individuals as much as 2,000 micrograms per day were required to normalize the blood selenium levels.

No signs of toxicity were observed in any patient—even in the autopsies of the 37 patients who were helped, but not cured by the therapy. It should also be pointed out that other antioxidant nutrients, vitamins A, C and E, were also used in the program.

It's time to cease debating the possibility the selenium helps cure cancer and move into large controlled clinical trials.

HEART DISEASE

It is not surprising that selenium is protective against heart disease. The main reason that Scott and Schwarz were studying selenium was that selenium deficiency in livestock caused heart and muscle disease. In cattle and sheep, selenium deficiency caused white muscle disease, which produced chalky striations of calcium in the muscles. In swine, selenium deficiency produced mulberry heart disease, which is named after the mulberry color of the heart tissue due to the blood infiltration. Another characteristic of mulberry heart disease is that when you lay a surgically removed mulberry-diseased heart on a table, it collapses. A healthy heart maintains a firm structure; selenium deficiency tends to weaken all muscle structure.

Livestock graze in a limited area and have a limited diet. It has always been thought that since people have a more diverse diet with foods coming from widely varied regions, man would never experience such gross selenium deficiency as seen in cattle and swine. Wrong. In 1981, the *New England Journal of Medicine* (304(21): 1304-1305) reported a case of cardiomyopathy in a young girl eating a diet essentially of hot dogs and cereal. After selenium supplementation, she improved dramatically and the disease was corrected.

But selenium's role in protection against heart disease is not limited to the health of the tissue or affected only by gross selenium deficiency; subclinical deficiency plays several roles in heart-related problems. In 1965, Dr. K. O. Godwin found that animals fed low-selenium diets developed abnormal electrocardiograms and blood pressure disturbances.

In *Supernutrition* (Dial Press, 1975; Pocket Books, 1977) I reported that a veterinary drug called Seletoc, a combination of selenium and vitamin E, had been in use since 1962 to successfully treat degenerative heart disease. In 1972, a variation of the formula, called Telsem, was reported to be 92 percent effective against recurring angina pectoris in dogs and was undergoing clinical trials in Mexico. The wide availability of selenium as a food supplement may have discouraged the completion of those trials. A drug has to produce a high profit margin to pay for the clinical trials, and the wide availability of inexpensive supplements removed the profit incentive.

However, research on the roles on selenium in protection against heart disease continued. In 1976, Drs. Ray Shamberger and Charles Willis of the Cleveland Clinic reported that persons living in low-selenium areas had three times more heart disease than those in selenium-rich areas. Tables 1 and 2 show this relationship in greater detail. Dr. Johan Bjorksten found

Table 1.
World heart disease rates versus selenium intake

Country	Selenium Intake micrograms/day	Coronary Heart Disease Rate
Finland	25	1009
USA	61	870
Canada	62	722
Ireland	75	722
Australia	76	867
Norway	82	602
Greece	92	236
Poland	94	301
Yugoslavia	99	232
Bulgaria	108	331

Selenium intake and coronary heart disease deaths per 100,000 in 55-to 64-year-old males in ten countries.

Source: Data with exception of Finland from Shamberger, R., Gunsch, M., Willis, C. and McCormack, L. 1975 *Trace Substances in Environmental Health* ix ed. D. Hemphill. Columbia: University of Mississippi Press, pp. 15–22. Author has corrected the Finnish figures to those used by Dr. Johan Bjorksten and Dr.Pekko Koivistoinen, head, Dept. of Food Chemistry and Technology, Univeristy of Helsinki.

Table 2.
U.S.A. heart disease death rates and selenium

Disease	Selenium levels			
	Very high	High	Medium	Low
MALES				
Coronary	774	818	893	962
Hypertensive	34	53	64	71
Cardiovascular Renal	1045	1149	1252	1308
Cerebrovascular	108	138	159	139
FEMALES				
Coronary	220	225	249	306
Hypertensive	27	39	47	53
Cardiovascular Renal	413	428	474	539
Cerebrovascular	89	94	109	104

Age-specific death rates per 100,000 for white males or females, age 55–65, 1959–1961. Selenium level classification, above 0.26 is very high, 0.10 to 0.25 is high. 0.06 to 0.09 is medium, and 0.01 to 0.05 is low.

Source: Shamberger, R. May 11–13, 1976. *Proceedings of the Symposium on Selenium-Tellurium in the Environment.* Univ. Notre Dame, p. 265.

that in Finnish counties having 0.1 parts per million (ppm) or more of selenium in the drinking water, the heart disease death rate in persons 15–64 was only one per 1730 persons. This compares to one heart disease death per 224 persons of the same age in counties where the drinking water contains 0.05 ppm or less of selenium.

In the mid-1970s, the relationship between selenium deficiency and high blood pressure was being pursued. One link between selenium deficiency and high blood pressure was a reduction in prostaglandin levels. Another link was that selenium detoxifies cadmium, which is known to elevate blood pressure.

A Discovery in China—Keshan Disease

China has a huge low-selenium belt running diagonally from the northeast to the southwest. A form of heart disease called Keshan disease is prevalent in this low-selenium area. Keshan disease resembles the mulberry heart disease described earlier.

The people most susceptible to this disease are children and women of child-bearing age.

A study of the effects of selenium supplements of Keshan disease was initiated in 1974. In Nianning County, selenium supplements were given to 4,510 children selected at random, while 3,985 others made up the control group receiving the placebo. The following year these two groups were increased to 6,709 and 5,445, respectively. The results were so dramatic that the control group was abolished in 1976 and all children were given selenium supplements. Thus, 99 percent of the children aged one to nine in four communes in the county participated in the clinical trial.

As reported in the *Chinese Medical Journal* and *Lancet*: "In 1974, of the 3,985 children in the control group, there were fifty-four cases of Keshan disease (1.35 percent), while only ten of the 4,510 selenium-supplemented children fell ill to the disease (0.22 percent). The difference in the morbidity rate between the two groups was highly significant.

"Again a significant difference was shown in the 1975 figures with fifty-two of 5,445 children in the control group (0.95 percent) and only seven of the 6,767 in the treated group (0.1 percent).

"As a result of these two years showed that oral administration of selenium had positive effects in the prevention of Keshan disease, all the children were given selenium supplements from 1976 on. In consequence, only four cases occurred out of the 12,579 children in 1976, further lowering the rate of 0.03 percent. *In 1977, there were no fresh cases among the 12,747 treated children.*" (*Chinese Medical Journal* 92 (7): 471-476, 1979; *Lancet*, Oct. 28, 1979, p. 890.)

Atherosclerosis and Common Forms of Heart Disease

Persons with low selenium blood levels develop significantly more heart disease than those with higher levels of selenium blood levels. In 1982, Dr. J. T. Salonen and his Finnish colleagues published an interesting prospective clinical study (*Lancet* 2:175). Blood samples were collected from approximately 11,000 Finns who were free of heart disease in 1972, and stored for analysis at a later date. During the next seven years 367 of these volunteers suffered a heart attack or died of heart disease. These subjects were matched with 367 volunteers of the same sex, age, lifestyle, etc., who remained free of heart disease, and the stored blood samples from these 724 individuals were retrieved and analyzed for selenium concentration.

The average selenium level in the blood from those who became stricken with heart disease during the seven-year period was significantly lower than the average blood selenium level from those who remained free of heart disease. A blood selenium level of less than 45 micrograms per liter was associated with a two- to threefold greater risk of heart disease as compared to subjects with higher blood selenium levels.

Another study demonstrated that there were actually fewer cholesterol deposits in the arteries of persons with higher levels of selenium in their blood. Drs. Julie Ann Moore, Robert Noiva and Ibert C. Wells of the Creighton University School of Medicine followed up the study led by Dr. Salonen by measuring the amount of selenium in the blood of patients about to have their arteries examined by arteriography (angiogram). In the 106 patients the extent of observed cholesterol deposits was inversely correlated with selenium level—the lower the selenium level, the more likely the presence of cholesterol deposits and the greater the extent.

The highest average selenium value (136 micrograms per liter) was found in those persons free of coronary blockage. Patients with the lowest average blood selenium level were found to have blockage of three coronary arteries. Patients with one or two blocked coronary arteries had intermediate blood selenium levels.

It is significant to know that selenium reduces heart disease incidence and death rate, yet scientists always want to know how and why. Part of the answer is that selenium is protective against heart disease by keeping arteries free of cholesterol deposits. But selenium also helps keep the blood "slippery." Since a heart attack is usually caused by a clot forming in a coronary artery which prevents oxygen from reaching the heart tissue serviced by that artery, having fewer cholesterol deposits on which clots can form, and "slippery" free-flowing blood, certainly diminishes the possibility of a clot forming.

Arteries produce a substance called prostacyclin which prevents blood clots. However, if oxidized fats are present in the blood, prostacyclin production is reduced, and the blood tends to clot. Selenium reduces the oxidation of fats in the blood and tissue, thereby helping to keep the prostacyclin level normal. Thus, the blood retains its normal—and appropriate—"slipperiness." This is different from anticoagulant drugs that can cause the blood to become so "slippery" that bleeding cannot be controlled or that spontaneous bleeding occurs.

Two studies published in 1984 examine this role of selenium. One is by Dr. N. W. Stead and colleagues as published in the *American Journal of Clinical Nutrition* (39:677) and the other is by Dr. R. Schiavon et al., in *Thrombosis Research* (34:389). The net effect was demonstrated in laboratory animals that had their coronary arteries tied off so as to produce the same effect as a blockage due to a clot in the coronary artery. Two teams of researchers found that selenium greatly reduced the damage to the heart caused by the stoppage of blood. (Koeler et al., *Kardiologiya* 25:9, 72-6, 1985 and Litvitskii et al., *Kardiologiya* 22:7, 94-8, 1982.)

Selenium has thus, been shown to be protective against heart disease by livestock animal studies, laboratory animal studies, epidemiological studies and human clinical studies. In addition, several mechanisms have been delineated through which selenium provides this protective action. These mechanisms include maintaining the integrity of heart and artery tissue, regulation of blood pressure, regulation of blood clotting and "slipperiness" and the reduction of plaque or cholesterol deposits in arteries.

ARTHRITIS

Arthritis is a multifactorial disease for which there is no agreed-upon cause or cure. Although the cause is not agreed upon, there is evidence that selenium relieves the symptoms. There is also evidence that selenium deficiency—or a general deficiency of the other antioxidant nutrients (vitamins A, C and E) plus selenium—contributes to the development of arthritis. The deficiency of the antioxidants allows the formation of excess free radicals which produce the pain and swelling of arthritis.

Superoxide dismutase (SOD), an enzyme that serves as an antioxidant, is also deficient in persons with arthritis. When additional SOD is injected into arthritic joints, significant reduction of swelling and pain is observed. There is evidence that the antioxidant enzyme glutathione peroxidase, which contains four atoms of selenium in every molecule, also reduces swelling and pain in arthritic joints.

Veterinarians have used a formulation containing 1,000 micrograms of selenium and 68 IU of vitamin E successfully for years in treating arthritic horses. The injections of SOD provide quicker results, but the selenium and vitamin E does work well. Now the same relief is being reported in people.

At the May 1980 meeting of selenium researchers, Norwegian scientists reported the beneficial results of selenium against arthritis: "In rheumatoid arthritis, it has been suggested that superoxide (free) radicals and lipoperoxides (also free radicals) can be generated in the tissues and accelerate the progression of the disease. Since selenium is a component of the protective enzyme glutathione peroxidase, we determined the blood levels of selenium in a group of twenty-three rheumatoid arthritis patients." (J. Aaseth et al., *Second International Symposium on Selenium in Biology and Medicine*, Texas Technical University, Lubbock, Texas, May 1980) The researchers found that the arthritis group did have depressed selenium levels compared to the reference group. At the same conference, Dr. E. Crary of Smyrna, Georgia had already treated patients having traumatic arthritis with selenium plus the antioxidant nutrients vitamins A, C and E, successfully relieving the pain in their traumatized joints.

In 1982, the British Arthritic Association conducted a three-month trial of formulation containing selenium plus vitamins A, C and E. The trial included some of the worst cases, and yet 64 percent reported considerable reduction in pain within the three months. Many continued the supplement and found continuing reduction in pain.

Among the patients was Mr. Charles Ware, 74, the British Arthritic Association's president, who developed arthritis of the hip after a fall during World War II. He told newspaper reporters, "I thought that I would never get rid of the pain. But now I have full movement of my hip and no pain whatever." The British Arthritic Association is now recommending selenium plus the antioxidant vitamins A, C and E to all its members.

Following newspaper accounts of this successful trial, the British magazine *Here's Health* distributed this same formulation of selenium plus the vitamins A, C and E to 1,000 volunteers. Replies to a follow-up questionnaire were received from 418 of the volunteers. Improvement was noted by 315 (75 percent).

A Danish study was published in 1985 that confirmed the 1980 Norwegian study. Blood selenium concentrations were measured in 87 patients with rheumatoid arthritis. The researchers headed by Dr. U. Tarp found significant differences in patients of the three distinct courses of the disease. The group having an active, disabling disease of long duration had a very reduced selenium level (65 mcg./1). The group with protracted but mild disease had a slightly reduced level (74 mcg./1). The group with mild disease of short duration had a slightly (but not statistically significant) reduced blood selenium level (76 mcg./1). The researchers concluded, "A low selenium level may thus be a further factor in the pathogenesis of rheumatoid arthritis." (*Scandinavian Journal of Rheumatology* 14:97-101, 1985)

Japanese researcher Dr. Masaru Kondo has found that treating persons with arthritis with 350 micrograms of selenium and 400 IU of vitamin E daily, plus injecting white blood cells from healthy people is very effective. All seven of his first patients improved dramatically, and five of the seven were essentially free of the disease by the time he wrote his report. (*Biological Trace Element Research* 7:195-198, May-June 1985)

When the white blood cell injections were given without the antioxidant supplements, only one of thirty rheumatoid arthritis patients obtained a complete remission. All patients had severe joint pains for over four years prior to the treatment, and their rheumatoid factor titer (RFT) was initially high (average 379). The five patients experiencing complete remission also had their RFT return to a normal of less than four. The remaining two patients had diminished joint pain and increased joint mobility.

FURTHER INFORMATION

This booklet has presented a sampling of the research that shows that selenium is protective against cancer, heart disease and arthritis. More details on this research plus the role of selenium in the protection against other diseases is found in my book *Selenium As Food and Medicine* (Keats Publishing).

Now that you have "sampled" SELENIUM —

Here is the best way to get more background information on this vital element — what therapy employing it has accomplished — and most importantly, how you can assure yourself of your body's needed supply of it.

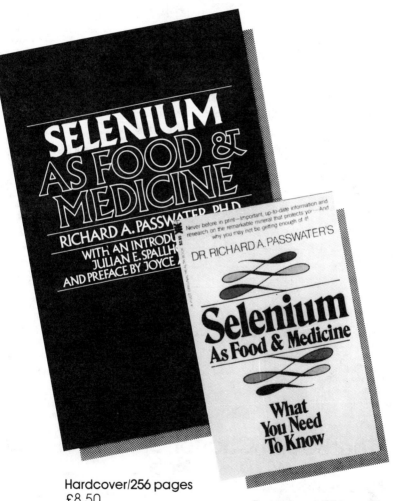

Hardcover/256 pages
£8.50

Paperback/256 pages
£2.30

Order Form

Please rush me the following books in quantities indicated:

__ copies **Selenium as Food and Medicine** (Hardcover £8.50)

__ copies **Selenium as Food and Medicine** (Paperback £2.30)

I enclose £_____(includes postage and handling) TOTAL £_____

OR charge my Access Card Account No. _____ Expires __/__/__

Your signature (if charged) _____

Your name (please print) _____

Address _____

Town _____ County _____ Post Code _____

At your favourite book store or health food store or use this page to order direct from the distributor. Please scotch tape — do not staple.
Cheque or Postal Order please. No cash.

Registered No: 1814017

From _____
_____
_____

Place
Stamp
Here

TO
The Health Charter Club (H.C.C. Ltd.)
8 Leatherhead Industrial Estate
Leatherhead
Surrey
KT22 7AG

Att'n Mail Order Department